Fibromyalgia

Fibromyalgia treatment including chronic pain relief, fibromyalgia diet and fitness

Copyright © 2014 by Wendy Owen (Natural Health Books).
All rights reserved worldwide. No part of this publication
may be replicated, redistributed, or given away in any
form without the prior written consent of the author/publisher
or the terms relayed to you herein.

Wendy Owen, Natural Health Books,
Greenbank, Qld, 4124, Australia

Table of Contents

Introduction 1

Traditional Approach to Treating Fibromyalgia 3

How to Diagnose Fibromyalgia 7

Central Sensitization 11

Stress 15

Fibromyalgia diet 19

Leaky Gut Syndrome 27

Hormones 31

Exercise 35

How to Improve Sleep With Fibromyalgia 39

What on Earth is Phytotherapy? 45

Does Fascia Matter? 49

Conclusion 53

Disclaimer 55

Introduction

Perhaps the most frustrating part of fibromyalgia for many people is that patients don't show any outward appearance of being unwell. "But you don't look sick..." is a statement that fibromyalgia patients hear quite often. Understandably it would make anyone want to rip their hair out! Suffering internally while appearing healthy on the outside is, unfortunately, part of the fibromyalgia sufferer's lot.

Most people with fibromyalgia are not looking for sympathy as much as understanding. They want their friends and family to understand why they can't come out to dinner when they look perfectly fine - "You were OK with going out last week so what's the matter now?"

Add this to the chronic pain that can come and go, the constant tiredness, the difficulty sleeping and the emotional seesaws and you may well understand why some fibromyalgia sufferers wonder if their life is over.

Heck no! There are people who have cured themselves from fibromyalgia. If they can, so can you! So let's get started. First up, a little bit about fibromyalgia, the traditional medical response and the difficulty of getting a proper diagnosis.

Never underestimate the body's ability to cure itself.

Traditional Approach to Treating Fibromyalgia

Doctors are usually fairly befuddled when recommending treatments for fibromyalgia. They adopt what we can call a scatter approach (throw enough stuff and something may stick). This is a risky approach when it comes to prescribing medication as many drugs have side effects and certain medications should not be taken together.

However doctors really don't have much choice when confronted with a patient who is experiencing pain, fatigue and sleep problems. Of course pain relief has to be the first consideration as pain contributes a lot to the other symptoms. Some fibromyalgia patients exist only on pain medication, handling the fatigue and sleep deprivation as best they can.

So what are the most common treatments being offered to fibromyalgia patients today and which are the most effective?

There are two medications that has now been specifically endorsed for use with fibromyalgia; *Lyrica* is perhaps the most well known, *Cymbalta* is actually an antidepressant. Doctors sometimes prescribe antidepressants as they can potentially address most of the symptoms with one medication. These can work well for some patients and not at all for others. These have not been recommended for long term use.

Cymbalta belongs to the family of antidepressants called *serotonin and noradrenaline reuptake inhibitors* (SNRIs). It is thought to have a beneficial effect on pain, sleep problems and of course depression. The pain relief would not be sufficient to take the pain away completely, so other pain medication would have to be taken.

Nausea, low energy and chronic sleep problems are some common side effects of Cymbalta. Interesting that this drug can cause the same health problems it seeks to treat.

Lyrica (Pregabalin) was the first drug officially approved for fibromyalgia and works by targeting pain centers in the brain. It works through the nerve centers that convey pain signals to the brain and lessens the frequency and intensity of these signals. Lyrica can help fibromyalgia sufferers with both pain and sleep difficulties, however it doesn't work for everyone.

Lyrica is actually an anticonvulsant drug usually prescribed for people with epilepsy. Are there side effects? Of course. The problem with Lyrica is that it can make depression worse and as depression is frequently a symptom of fibromyalgia, this can be a huge concern. Only accept a recommendation for Lyrica if you have no symptoms of depression!

Lyrica can also increase *creatinine kinase* levels in the blood, potentially leading to muscle pain – not exactly what you need with Fibromyalgia.

In spite of the above caveats, Lyrica can really help many people with fibromyalgia.

Savella is another medication that has recently been put forward as a fibromyalgia treatment. Savella is also an SNRI and can reduce pain levels in fibromyalgia. Side effects are similar to those of other SNRIs. Always talk to your doctor before taking any of the above medications, especially if you are already on any other medication, including herbal remedies. Pregnant or breast feeding women need to take special care before commencing any medication, so always tell your doctor if you are pregnant or are breast feeding.

These are the typically prescribed medications for fibromyalgia. Of course over the counter (OTC) pain meds are often taken as well as, or in place of, the above. As always, speak to your doctor before making any changes to your medications.

How to Diagnose Fibromyalgia

Fibromyalgia is a debilitating and painful disease that affects over ten million people in the US and many millions more worldwide. It is one of the least understood diseases in medical circles and therefore one of the hardest to diagnose.

If you have been through this process, you would probably already know how difficult it is to get a concrete diagnosis of fibromyalgia. In fact fibromyalgia was only recognized as a disease in its own right in 1990 by a Dr Frederick Wolfe. Despite this however, there are still those in the medical community that are not sold on the fact that fibromyalgia is a real complaint, despite it being recognized by the American College of Rheumatology. Most people seeking a diagnosis for their symptoms have to go from doctor to doctor to find an answer and the diagnosis can take from months to years.

The reason why diagnosis is so difficult is because there are many different aspects to the disease – hence the name "fibromyalgia syndrome". The main ones that most people recognize are widespread pain and ongoing fatigue and these can be symptomatic of several other diseases, for instance rheumatoid arthritis and chronic fatigue syndrome. There are no blood tests that can confirm the disease; so what does constitute a diagnosis of fibromyalgia?

A classic diagnosis consists of the patient experiencing pain in at least eleven of eighteen points in the body as set out by the American College of Rheumatology (ACR).

The reason there needs to be at least 11 points is that there may be other causes for pain in these areas, such as arthritis or poor posture. Looking at these points makes it understandable when a person with fibromyalgia says they "hurt all over!"

We'll look at these points starting from the top of the body:

1. The back of the neck, where the base of the skull and the neck meet.
2. The front of the neck above the collarbone, on both sides of the throat
3. The front of the body, a couple of inches below the collarbone and either side of the breast bone.
4. Upper back, between the shoulder and the bottom of the neck
5. Around the shoulder blades
6. On the outer forearms near the elbow crease, toward the outer arm
7. Lower back towards the top of the buttocks
8. In the hips, just between buttocks and thigh muscles
9. Inside the knee pads

If a patient experiences pain when pressure is applied to these points (allodynia) and also experiences symptoms of fatigue and perhaps sleep disturbances, then they are said to have fibromyalgia. The symptoms also have to have been present for a period of three months or longer.

There are other symptoms that can be present in a person with fibromyalgia, these are stiffness in the joints, cognitive dysfunction (brain fog), difficulty when swallowing, digestive problems and depression. Not all those with fibromyalgia experience the full range of symptoms and some people have symptoms that come and go and are worse at some times than others.

The great majority of fibromyalgia sufferers are women at a ratio of almost 10 to 1, a fact that still puzzles the medical community and research on this is ongoing. This does seem to indicate, however that hormones play a role in this disease.

Stress

The medical community is not convinced that stress is a risk factor for fibromyalgia , but evidence is mounting that stress is indeed a major cause. According to Dr Mehmet Oz MD, "Stress causes changes in brain chemicals, and these are actually pretty similar to the changes we see in people with fibromyalgia."

If we can think of fibromyalgia as an energy crisis where the disease is consuming more energy than the body can make, then stress can indeed be a risk factor as it certainly drains our energy as much, if not more, than poor nutrition or the common cold. Stress is a leading cause of many diseases and it stands to reason that fibromyalgia is just another one.

The obvious answer is to reduce stress in our daily lives, but this is sometimes not as simple as doing thirty minutes of meditation or a yoga class twice a week, even though these do sometimes help temporarily! We may not be able to change stressful situations, especially if they're tied in with our jobs or families. However there are ways we can reduce stress beyond the usual advice and we'll look at that in a further chapter.

Age, gender, hormones and viruses also have a role to play when it comes to fibromyalgia.

Please understand that I am not trying to denigrate doctors or the medical profession in general. They are great at what they do. They have been trained in a set of criteria and have limited knowledge outside of it. Not their fault! Having said that, there are doctors who have an open mind to alternative ideas and therapies. If you find one of these gems, hold onto them with both hands. They're not very easy to find but they do exist, so don't stop looking for one.

I have spoken and worked with many people who have fibromyalgia, so I'm here to tell you that there is hope of getting rid of this disease as I know at least one person who is totally symptom free. Others have had their condition improve to the point where it mostly doesn't bother them at all.

There are many so called "causes" for fibromyalgia. These included stress, poor nutrition, hormonal imbalance (thyroid and adrenal dysfunction), infections and toxins. We will be examining all these and more to ensure by the time you have finished this book, you will know what you can do to get this horrible disease under control or, better still, get rid of it completely.

Are you ready????

Central Sensitization

Have you ever wondered why two people with the same complaint experience different levels of pain? A good example of this is a "bulging" disc in the spine. Many older people have this complaint and yet some feel no pain whatsoever, while others experience pain on a daily basis and can't get through the day with pain relief medication.

The answer lies in the central nervous system and the way it processes pain. Our brains contain pain receptors called neurons which cause us to feel pain. This is designed for our safety as in the example of little Johnny putting his hand on a hot stove. The immediate signal sent to his hand is pain and Johnny's reflexes cause him to pull his hand away very quickly! Johnny has also established a subconscious "pain memory", so he never puts his hand on the stove again.

Now this is fine for isolated emergencies, but when it comes to chronic pain, the continuous pain signals stimulate the brain neurons causing them to develop a constant and permanent pain memory, thus training them to become more sensitive to pain and overreact to pain signals. This is known as *Central Sensitization*.

Scientists have conducted brain imaging on people with fibromyalgia and arthritis who suffer with chronic pain. They found definite evidence that the brains of chronic pain sufferers behaved differently in an area called the *insula cortex* among other areas. What this means to us is that fibromyalgia patients have a lower pain threshold than most other people.

Without going too far into the science, Levels of *Substance P* (a neurotransmitter that allows nerve cells to communicate with one another) is increased in chronic pain patients, while levels of calming neurotransmitter *serotonin* and the amino acid *tryptophan* are decreased. This would also explain the sleep difficulties people experience in fibromyalgia, since serotonin is necessary for good sleep and feelings of calm.

Substance P's main function is to transmit pain messages, so anything that can decrease the level of Substance P in fibromyalgia sufferers, can potentially decrease the level of pain they experience.

Medical science has come up with an answer to decreasing Substance P and that is *Capsaicin cream.*

Capsaicin cream is applied topically, which means it is rubbed into a painful area and, with time, will decease the level of pain felt in that area.

Capsaicin cream is made from the chilli plant and it is very hot. When applying, make sure you wash your hands well afterward with soap to make sure all the cream is removed. The cream may burn the skin where it is applied initially, but this effect should lessen in a week or so.

Capsaicin cream will take time to work – sometimes up to a month. It does provide relief, however treatment must be continued indefinitely, or the effect will wear off.

Is there anything else we can do to reduce Substance P levels? Read on...

Substance P is said to increase with stress, whether physical or emotional. You can see how this creates a nasty vicious cycle, more pain – more stress – more substance P! There are a couple of supplements we can take to help decrease the effects of stress and Substance P and help breakdown the pain cycle:

Serotonin – The best way to boost your serotonin levels is by taking a precursor such as *tryptophan* or *5-HTP*. Both can be converted into serotonin. Of the two, 5HTP is probably the more effective. It can pass through the blood/brain barrier very quickly and be converted into serotonin. Aim for a good quality, sustained release brand and follow the dosage on the label. Serotonin will help lower pain levels, improve sleep and as a bonus, will ease carbohydrate cravings.

Quercetin – This is a potent anti-oxidant which is beneficial for good health. It is said to help remove Substance P from nerves. It also offers protection against stress by suppressing the enzyme needed for cortisol release. You can obtain quercetin naturally from foods, such as fruits and vegetables (berries, grapes, green tea and citrus fruits), but for a quick boost, a supplement is recommended. Check with your doctor before taking quercetin as it can react with other medications.

Exercise can also significantly decrease the effects of Substance P and is beneficial for people with fibromyalgia. Stretching will also help. Just move! It doesn't matter how slowly you start, every little bit will help.

Massage can decrease Substance P levels, at least temporarily and also has a beneficial effect on stress.

All the above can help decrease Substance P on a temporary basis, but *is it possible to get rid of it permanently?*

I believe that it is. Using a process called *EFT*, people have been able to lower substance P and significantly reduce their pain levels. EFT (Emotional Freedom Technique) can be used directly on chronic pain, insomnia and stress. I have been into this in detail in the Stress chapter. EFT for fibromyalgia is particularly helpful due to the combination of symptoms. It seems to work best when the symptoms are addressed separately rather than as a whole.

Find out more about EFT here:- http://www.eftuniverse.com/

Stress

Opinions differ widely, but more and more evidence is pointing to stress as a cause of fibromyalgia. There may be many triggers, for instance accidents, surgery and emotional or physical trauma, just to name a few, but what all these triggers have in common is they all cause stress in the body. Physical stress more often than not, will lead to emotional stress compounding the effects.

Why the body responds in such a way, no-one really knows. Fibromyalgia is not the only result of stress, there are many diseases such as cancer, insomnia, depression, viruses, circulation and heart disease, diabetes and other auto-immune diseases that are now thought to be caused by stress.

The main reason for this is that stress and its cousins anxiety and worry can disable the immune system to such a degree that it can no longer protect us from germs and viruses. The immune system can also turn on the body leading to auto immune diseases such as rheumatoid arthritis. There is no disease on the planet than can't be relieved to some extent by reducing stress.

Chronic stress can be a killer, so how do we combat it?

Recognize what causes stress in your life. What freaks one person out may just cause another to shrug and smile - we are all different and you really need to know what's causing stress and anxiety in your own life.

Once you know this, then you can work at eliminating as much stress as possible. Of course you won't be able to get rid of it all; your stress may be caused by your job or your family. In cases where you can't, or don't want to, change your situation, you need to learn how to manage it.

OK how to manage stress?

Meditation

Typical advice on stress management has never done much for me, especially when it comes to meditation. Yes, I know meditation is the answer to just about everything according to the health gurus. It decreases cortisol levels, lowers blood pressure, improves sleep, makes you look younger, makes you rich (joke!), but I just can't get the hang of it. I have an unlimited number of guided meditation CDs and MP3s, but I still can't get any benefit out of it.

I'm not trying to put anyone off starting meditation, some things work better for some people. I know people who meditate daily and swear by it. If you can discipline your mind and make it work for you, you will benefit by being able to relax at will.

Deep breathing

This is easy, free and works very well. There are many deep breathing exercises that you can try, but simply breathing deeply into the diaphragm and breathing out slowly will do the trick. Make sure your are filling the bottom of the lungs as you do this - (your stomach will push out). Breathing in this way is called belly breathing and it engages the parasympathetic nervous system which calms you down if practiced for five minutes or longer.

Exercise

This works for me, just about any exercise does the trick. Although yoga is most often recommended for relaxation, walking, swimming or doing an exercise class works just as well. I think it's the fact that exercise removes us from the source of stress and forces us to think about something else. It also increases circulation and oxygen intake which refreshes the whole body.

Energy therapy

Now I know a few of you are going to tune out around about now – **please don't**. This flat out works, whether you believe in it or not. The therapy I'm recommending is called EFT, short for Emotional Freedom Technique.

EFT used to be considered useful for emotional distress, but it's since been discovered that it will work on physical ailments too. This could possibly be because all physical conditions have an emotional component, but no-one really knows. Just the fact that it works is enough for most people!

EFT has been described as "acupuncture without needles". It consists of tapping on certain energy meridian points on the body to balance the "Qi" (energy that flows through the body). EFT is credited with successfully treating many diseases that conventional medicine can't touch. It is wonderful for relieving stress and – of most interest to fibromyalgia sufferers, relieving pain. EFT has proved successful on migraine headaches, back pain, arthritis pain, nerve pain and of course fibromyalgia. Here is a link to the EFT website where you can access a free manual and read countless articles on different uses for EFT.

http://www.eftuniverse.com/

Please do this for yourself – just give it a try; there is nothing to lose. EFT is completely harmless and free to use. I have used it many times for pain relief and for quitting smoking. Some issues will take longer to heal than others and may require a bit of persistence. I will say this upfront – pain relief can take quite a while before you see results. If you are persistent and keep chipping away at the different aspects as they arise, you should notice a difference in time.

Stress can be dealt with quite quickly with EFT, however it may come back unless you address the cause of the stress. Of course you can do also do this with EFT.

Does EFT heal the body? Not strictly speaking, but it will clear the way for the body to heal itself. It can also deal with limiting beliefs which can stop us from succeeding in any area of life. If you suffer from depression, EFT can help here too as it is wonderful for dealing with negative thoughts and emotions. EFT has been used to treat post traumatic stress disorder in Vietnam vets with spectacular results.

OK, I'll stop prattling on now. Hopefully I've awakened enough interest for you to just go and take a peek :)

Fibromyalgia diet

Although the medical fraternity doesn't place much emphasis on diet as it relates to fibromyalgia, what you eat is of supreme importance when it comes to this disease.

If you have fibromyalgia, something in your body is broken. Fibromyalgia can't be conveniently blamed on a bad diet – there can be so many different causes, but it will certainly need a good diet to fix it! While most people can get away with the odd meal of junk food without their health suffering too much, fibromyalgia sufferers don't have that luxury.

Fear not though. The eating plan necessary to overturn fibromyalgia doesn't have to be followed for the rest of your life. It can, and should be, modified and tweaked so it suits your tastes while remaining as healthy as possible. The upside to this of course is a knowledge of what to put, and what not to put, into your body for maximum health and energy and even pain relief.

Nutrition 101

Eating whole, fresh organic foods (fruits, vegetables, and high-quality fats and protein) is the best way to nourish your body and to reverse disease. As I said in the introduction, the body never stops trying to heal itself, it just needs the right tools. Food is one of the most important tools for disease reversal.

If you are under a lot of stress, it's a good idea to take a pharmaceutical grade multivitamin and mineral complex. Your muscles, nervous system, adrenal glands, immune system and your body needs proper nutrition for the healing process to take place.

A lot of people say they can't afford organic vegetables. To them I say "It's cheaper than a lifetime of pharmaceutical drugs!" There is also another option – grow your own! That way you can ensure that they contain no chemical pesticides or fertilizers and that the soil they grow in is rich and of good quality.

Before beginning any new eating plan, it's a great idea to detoxify the body to get rid of built up chemicals, heavy metals and other parasites that may be contributing to your condition. Although the body does quite a good job of detoxifying itself, the chemicals in food, in the home and even in the environment these days, can build up to dangerous levels even in the most healthy individuals. In people with fibromyalgia, these toxins must be purged from the body for any improvement to have a chance.

This is especially important if you suffer with any type of digestive issues such as constipation, irritable bowel, skin problems, bloating or diarrhea. If you have been trying to lose weight without success, this too could be caused by toxic waste. Here's how to rid the body of toxins and ensure maximum absorption of all the nutrition from our food and supplements.

First and most important is water. Most of us and walking around dehydrated without even realizing it. If you wait until you're thirsty before having a drink, then your body is sending a distress signal. Drink at least two liters a day. The best way I have found to do this is to keep your bottle or glass near you always and sip throughout the day. Makes sure you use steel or glass bottles instead of plastic. Your digestion will improve dramatically when you increase your water intake.

Green tea can be substituted for some of the water especially in the colder weather. Don't drink sodas or flavored mineral waters. Give coffee and black tea a miss for a while until after the detox as they are high in caffeine.

Cut out ALL processed food. Any food that comes in a box or packet is processed and is pretty much devoid of nutrition. For example breakfast cereals, muesli bars, potato or corn chips, biscuits, cakes... you get the idea. Eat whole foods such as grass fed meats, chicken, fresh fish (check the mercury levels). Include different types of vegetables and plenty of high fiber foods like whole grain breads, pasta and brown rice. Avoid white flour, white bread and any food that contains artificial coloring, artificial flavoring or chemical preservatives. These are all toxic substances which will lodge in your fat tissues and cause not just digestive issues, but potential disease and chronic pain.

Cut out dairy foods for a few weeks while your body is detoxing. Dairy allergies or intolerances are very common and you may feel significantly better without it. There are a couple of exceptions, plain yoghurt and whey powder are both dairy based, but healthy foods.

Butter is a good fat, despite what you may have heard to the contrary. It is far better for you than margarine, which is a horrible toxic food. Although butter falls under the dairy label, it is really a fat and contains little milk protein.

Eggs are a quality food and contrary to myth, will not raise your cholesterol levels. Eat them instead of cheese for a quick protein fix.

Don't eat late at night. Make dinner your last food for the day. This gives your digestive system time to process what you've eaten. Never go to bed on a full stomach.

A couple of supplements to help with your detox....

Chlorella – chlorella is invaluable during a detox as it will help remove toxins from the body. It is potent enough to even remove heavy metals like mercury as well as pesticides. Chlorella is considered a superfood as it promotes growth and repair of the body's tissues as well as being a rich source of vitamins and minerals.

When purchasing chlorella, be sure to get a brand where the outer cell wall has been broken down, as it is very tough and may not break down in the body. Start slowly with chlorella to allow your body time to build up tolerance.

Modified Citrus Pectin (MCP) – this is a fruit pectin that has been altered to be digestible by the human body. It is a powerful detoxer to the point where it can remove heavy metals from the blood stream and body tissues. MCP promotes cellular health and is sometimes used when extreme measures to remove heavy metals, like chelation, are not possible.

After making these changes, you should notice some changes in your digestion within a week or so. You may even start to feel worse before you feel better, but that's just your body cleaning out and adjusting. If there's no improvement in thirty days, try cutting out gluten. This is found in bread and all wheat products, rye, pasta, gravy mixes and in many packaged foods. Even some bottled sauces contain gluten.

If removing gluten from your diet helps you to feel better then you may have a gluten sensitivity. This may not mean you will never be able to eat gluten again, simply that you need to give your digestive system a rest from it for a while. After your detox, try adding gluten foods one by one and see how your body reacts.

Sometimes just doing the above can cut your pain levels down significantly. If this is the case for you, be aware when adding potential allergens such as wheat and dairy back into your diet. Add them one at a time and give them two to three days for any symptoms to appear.

After your detox, try to stick to your food plan as much as possible. Eating junk, especially sugar and drinking soda will never do anything for you. You can actually live a much better quality of life without these "foods".

Supplements

There are certain supplements which benefit people with fibromyalgia. I have listed these below:

B-complex vitamins – These are beneficial for energy, boosting immunity, nerve health, and good brain function. Try and find a whole food source of B-complex – not the chemical variety.

Magnesium - maybe the most important mineral for those with F. Magnesium is not easily absorbed by the body so make sure you digestion is in tip-top health. Good magnesium sources are citrate, glycinate, taurate and theonate. Magnesium oxide is not well absorbed, so don't waste your money on it. Magnesium chloride comes in liquid form and can be rubbed on the body where it is absorbed into the bloodstream through the skin.

A lot of people in the US are deficient in magnesium – around 80%. Deficiency can cause muscle tightness and pain as well as a range of other health issues so make sure you're getting enough. Food rich in magnesium are almond, flax-seed, whey, pumpkin seeds, sunflower seed and spinach. If you have F, it's a great idea to also take a supplement.

Sam-E – Sam E is an enzyme used by the body to produce the neurotransmitters serotonin and dopamine, which tend to be low in people with fibromyalgia. Sam-E can alleviate F symptoms such as pain and depression.

Iodine – This is necessary for thyroid health and has been found to be very low in those with fibromyalgia. See more about thyroid health in the chapter on hormones.

CoQ10 - breaks down food to form ATP to produce energy. Great for chronic fatigue, it's best taken with meals containing fat. Give CoQ10 a few weeks before seeing results.

L-Carnitine – helps to lessen pain and boosts the mood of F sufferers. It also increases energy by breaking down fat.

I hope I have provided enough material in this chapter to help kick start your journey towards greater health and less pain. Dietary solutions are not drugs; they are far safer, but take a little while longer to work.

Leaky Gut Syndrome

What is a leaky gut and why should I care?

Leaky gut is a condition in which the walls of the small intestine become irritated, allowing small gaps to form in the cells of the wall barrier. This allow toxins, undigested food particles, fungi, parasites, bacteria and other waste matter to leak through into the bloodstream.

Leaky gut in a very common condition which can cause a whole range of health complaints including auto-immune system diseases, chronic fatigue system and fibromyalgia – just to name a few.

Leaky gut can also prevent nutrients from being absorbed by the intestines and can cause nutritional deficiencies, particularly mineral deficiencies, as these are typically hard for the body to absorb. This could be one reason why most fibromyalgia sufferers have a lack of magnesium, even if their intake of magnesium is adequate. Lack of magnesium is known to cause tightness and pain in the muscles. There is a work-around for this – please see the chapter on diet.

Leaky gut is thought to be caused by overuse of antibiotics and also from the use of non steroidal anti inflammatory drugs (NSAIDs). NDAIDs are often taken for pain in diseases such as rheumatoid arthritis (Aleve, Motrin) or for a simple headache (Aspirin). NSAIDs are notorious for inflaming the intestinal walls, which eventually leads to leakage and even bleeding.

Antibiotics cause leaky gut more indirectly. They destroy beneficial bacteria which usually transform dangerous toxins, wastes and bile salts before they can do damage. Left untreated, these substances can cause damage to the colon preventing healthy nutrients from being absorbed. Inflammation can occur either affecting the joints (rheumatoid arthritis) or the muscles (fibromyalgia).

Liver damage can also result from these parasites, as it tries vainly to remove them from the body. The immune system struggles to cope and ultimately gives up the fight, leading to auto immune system diseases. The body systems are very complex and putting stress on any part of the system, will eventually result in damage to the whole.

Antibiotics can also cause Candida, a yeast overgrowth in the intestines. Candida can lead to shrinkage of the cells in the intestinal wall directly causing leaky gut.

Certain foods can also cause or exacerbate leaky gut. Sugar and processed foods are notorious for this and wheat can also cause problems in certain people. Too much alcohol can irritate the gut. Stress can also add to the burden.

Now we know what causes leaky gut, what steps can we take to cure it?

The first step is to improve our diet and remove foods which place a load on the gut. This includes, sugar, processed foods, wheat (gluten) and other grains, alcohol, sodas and vegetable oils (soybean, canola, cottonseed, corn and sunflower). This list doesn't include everything that may irritate the gut, but it's a great start. If you are intolerant to milk, cut all dairy out too.

Start a course of probiotics and digestive enzymes. Digestive enzymes do exactly what they say, help with digestion. This means there will be less undigested food particles to leak out of the gut.

Probiotics will help re-instate healthy bacteria back into the gut. This is essential for intestinal health. Probiotics support white blood cell function. These are natural killer cells that help to combat viruses or other foreign matter in the gut. Probiotics can also help soothe the inflammation response in the intestinal walls. Probiotics help to improve immune function which can benefit those with fibromyalgia. Some yogurts contain probiotics, but to ensure you are getting enough, so supplementing is best.

Aloe Vera juice has healing properties that can help heal and soothe the intestinal wall. Mix with lemon juice for an alkalizing benefit.

Glutamine can help heal leaky gut. It's an amino acid that will promote intestinal health and prevent carbohydrate cravings. Glutamine is necessary for proper lymphocyte function which is beneficial for those with immune issues. Start with 3000 mg daily and increase slowly. Glutamine is a safe supplement and required in fairly high doses for healing a leaky gut.

Get excess stress out of your life. See the chapter on stress for ways to do this.

Don't overeat and make sure you eat slowly and chew each mouthful thoroughly. This will help your digestion.

If you have tried all the above and see no improvement, try

aggressively cutting chemicals out of your life (it's a good idea to do this anyway). Use cosmetics with only natural ingredients and deodorant with no aluminum. Use natural cleaning products with no harsh chemical ingredients. While it's impossible to completely remove all chemicals from our lifestyles, we can help restore the balance by being aware of everything we use. While this can be tedious to start with, eventually it will become a habit and your health will reap the benefits.

Detoxify your body (see the section on diet for how to do this) Also take chlorella or modified citrus pectin to extract heavy metals from your tissues.

Hormones

Your hormones are the messengers of the body. The hypothalamus acts as command central sending messages to your thyroid gland and your adrenals among others. Research suggests that people with fibromyalgia may have disruptions in hormone sequences. This could be due to genetics as well as environmental and psychological stress.

For instance, there is a proven link between fibromyalgia and poor thyroid function. So what is the thyroid and how can we make it perform better?

The thyroid is an endocrine gland situated in the neck. It's your main gland for energy, metabolism and overall health. It produces thyroid hormones which control hundreds of functions in the body. The thyroid communicates with other glands in the body, keeping all the cells working properly. If thyroid hormone levels are low, this disrupts many bodily functions, including energy production.

How do I know when my thyroid hormone levels are low?

There are tests that your doctor can perform, but these are not very reliable. However there are certain symptoms that can indicate poor thyroid function. If you have several or all of the symptoms below, chances are your thyroid is not performing at its best.

- Severe fatigue, especially in the afternoon
- Rough dry skin and/or hair

- Sensitivity to cold and difficulty sweating even when warm
- Hair loss
- Weight gain, especially if not linked to diet
- Depression
- Brittle nails
- Constipation
- Stiff joints
- Muscles tightness

What can cause poor thyroid function?

Stress and Adrenal Function – Stress is one of the worst thyroid offenders. Your thyroid function is intimately tied to your adrenal function, which is intimately affected by how you handle stress.

Toxins and chemicals in the atmosphere or in food.

Gluten sensitivity, or other food intolerances.

Lack of iodine - Iodine used to be plentiful in our food supply, however it has diminished over recent years due to less use of iodine in agriculture. It has been speculated that at least 50% of the population could be iodine deficient leading to several diseases, one of which is hypothyroidism. We also have over-exposure to toxic competing halogens such as bromine, fluorine and chlorine. These occupy the iodine receptors in the body, meaning less iodine is absorbed.

If you have any of the symptoms of an under-active thyroid, make sure you increase your iodine levels. Here's how:

- Make sure your drinking water is fluoride free
- Use iodized salt
- Avoid sodas
- Avoid plastic containers for storing food
- Eat organic fruits and vegetables, this lessens your exposure to pesticides
- Use natural skincare products. Chemicals are absorbed through the skin
- Eat more fish. Just make sure it's mercury free

It's much safer to get your iodine naturally rather than from supplements, as too much iodine can be as harmful as too little.

There are many similarities between fibromyalgia and an underactive thyroid. A lot of the symptoms are similar, especially fatigue, brain fog and depression. Some people with thyroid conditions do experience muscle and joint pain, it usually isn't as severe as it is in a person who has fibromyalgia though.

The adrenal glands are affected in those with both conditions. Most people with fibromyalgia and thyroid-related conditions have unbalanced hormones.

Both require lifestyle changes for any improvement to take place.

It is tempting, but not realistic to conclude that thyroid conditions can cause fibromyalgia, however the link is definitely there.

Most chronic pain is just one symptom of a much greater problem, which accounts for the majority of patients' illnesses. The problem is hypothyroidism.

Dr Mark Starr - Hypothyroidism Type 2: The Epidemic
So it seems that at least one eminent doctor thinks that hypothyroidism could contribute to fibromyalgia and other chronic pain conditions. It would seem worthwhile then to make sure your thyroid is functioning optimally!

Exercise

People with fibromyalgia often dislike exercise as it causes them pain. They also argue that they are too tired to do any exercise. This is perfectly understandable, but exercise is so beneficial for fibromyalgia that it is worth persevering. Lack of exercise will lead to muscle de-conditioning and increase fatigue and pain.

Here are the best exercises that will help fibromyalgia without causing excess pain.

Slow and steady wins the race! Nowhere is this more applicable than when it comes to fibromyalgia. Avoid fast, jerky movements that can jar the body and cause pain. In my opinion, aquarobics is one of the best exercises for those with fibromyalgia as any movements are always slowed underwater. Also the warm water has a beneficial and relaxing effect on muscles.

If you join an aquarobics class, don't feel that you have to keep up. There will be people there that are probably younger and fitter than you, so just move gently and take things at your own pace. Make sure the water is warm before you get in as cold water can shock the muscles and make them stiffer.

Stationary bike. This is probably better than a real bike because you can go at your own pace, you don't have to go uphill and you don't get attacked by dogs! Start slowly and work up gradually to a longer distance at higher speeds. Don't try and break the land speed record though, there are no medals for this!

Plain old walking is fine. Our bodies were made for walking and it can't do any harm. Invest in the best quality walking shoes your budget will allow and stop often if you're feeling tired. As with anything, start slowly and build up gradually to a faster pace and longer distances.

Low impact aerobics can be very beneficial because there is minimal stress on muscles and joints and enough variety to exercise all parts of the body. Most good classes will offer a low impact variation on any move, so make sure the class you choose offers this.

Stretching is great for building muscles. This surprises some people, as stretching seems like a tame activity when compared to more active exercises such as jogging. Stretching is probably best combined with low impact aerobics as it has little heart/lung benefits on its own.

Stretching also increases flexibility of the muscles, fascia, tendons and even scar tissue. It can increase energy, decrease stress and enhance sleep

Not recommended—

Running. Running puts significant stress on the body. Each time your feet touch the ground it will jolt your muscles and joints. Running used to be considered a healthy exercise, but now a lot of health experts are not recommending it, even for healthy folk. It can cause heart problems.

Weight training. It is too easy to injure yourself working with weights. If you're concerned about maintaining muscle density, stretching will work just as well.

Any exercise with a lot of repetitive movements. This tends to cause more muscle pain in those with fibromyalgia. Stay with exercises with a whole range of motion that work out the whole body.

Zumba. I tried this once and it nearly killed me.....

There is no need to exercise every day, allow at least a day in between to give your muscles rest and repair time.

Some people with fibromyalgia experience low blood pressure. This can cause dizziness during or after exercise. To combat this, put some salt in your drinking water. This has dual benefits - it tends to increase blood pressure and will keep water in your bloodstream longer which prevents dehydration.

Don't forget to drink plenty of water during and after exercise.

How to Improve Sleep With Fibromyalgia

Most people with fibromyalgia (around 80%) also suffer with sleep disturbances. This is a vicious cycle in which pain is preventing sleep and lack of sleep is exacerbating pain. If sleep can be improved, then pain levels also tend to be lower, so it's vital to try and improve sleep by what ever means we can get hold of.

Sleep disturbances in those with fibromyalgia vary from the mundane, such as inability to fall asleep, early awakening etc, to the exotic – slow sleep disturbance.

Slow sleep, also known as deep sleep or more recently N3, is the most restorative phase of sleep. During the stages of deep sleep, the brain exhibits very slow brainwaves. These are known as theta and delta waves. When we are awake during the day, our brains emit the faster beta type brainwaves, alternating with slightly slower alpha waves. Alpha waves are associated with a relaxed awake state, whereas beta waves are found when the brain is highly alert.

People with fibromyalgia often report that their sleep doesn't refresh them. When waking from several hours sleep, they still feel tired and drained. This is typical of deep sleep deprivation and is the main reason why people with fibromyalgia experience chronic fatigue and "fibro fog" which is a nickname for the inability to focus and concentrate.

A normal sleep cycle consists of several stages and people cycle between light sleep, deep sleep and REM (dreaming) sleep every ninety minutes or so. During deep sleep, the brain slows down to theta and delta waves and the body repairs and restores itself. During this restorative phase, human growth hormone (HGH) is released which repairs all cells in the body including the muscles. Brain function and memory is also refreshed and events from short term memory get put into long term memory.

People with fibromyalgia seem to experience an interrupted deep sleep phase in which faster alpha waves are mixed in with theta and delta waves. This disruption impairs the restoration of the body and brain and the release of HGH quite significantly, leaving those with fibromyalgia tired and unable to function normally. It would also have a worsening effect on pain levels throughout the body.

Although sleep medication is often prescribed for people with fibromyalgia, it doesn't have much beneficial effect on deep sleep interruptions, although it can be helpful for those who have trouble falling asleep. The fibromyalgia medication *Lyrica*, however, seems to have a beneficial effect on deep sleep and therefore pain levels. Unfortunately Lyrica has a laundry list of side effects which can be lessened by starting on a low dose and increasing it gradually.

What causes these interruptions in the deep sleep cycle? Some researchers thinks it's simply the constant pain that disturbs the delta waves, but others theorize that it may be a chemical imbalance in the brain. The levels of the neurotransmitters serotonin, dopamine and norepinephrine and the hormone cortisol seem to be out of whack.

There is a lower level of serotonin in people with fibromyalgia which would have an effect both on sleep and on pain levels.

Stress levels may also play a part in the interruption of the deep sleep cycle. A stressed body will stay in what's known as "fight or flight" mode, meaning it's always on the alert for danger. Failure to turn off the fight or flight response prior to sleep may lead to impaired deep sleep and less quality sleep in general.

So how can people with fibromyalgia improve their sleep? First it's important to practice good sleep hygiene. This is simply done by following the instructions below.

Exercise every day if possible with gentle activities such as swimming yoga or walking. This will help ease fibromyalgia symptoms as well as improving sleep.

Don't spend too long in bed. If you wake up early in the morning, get up and start your day. This will tell the subconscious mind that bed means sleep.

Keep a sleep diary. Each morning write down how you slept the night before and note any situations that may have interfered with your sleep. Reviewing your diary over a period of time may give you valuable insights into your sleep problems.

Use relaxation therapies. Deep breathing, meditation, massage, progressive muscle relaxation and other relaxation techniques are all helpful to managing the symptoms of fibromyalgia and increasing restful sleep.

Don't nap during the day. If you must, keep naps to under twenty minutes. Otherwise you may go into deep sleep which will keep you awake later that night.

Get up at the same time every morning no matter what. Yes even on weekends! You will be surprised how this will help improve your sleep.

Interruptions of the deep sleep phase may be improved by increasing serotonin levels. Here are some ways of achieving this :

Get sunlight into your eyes during the day – the earlier the better. This rapidly increases serotonin production. Later in the evening the body will convert this into melatonin (your body-clock hormone), helping improve the quality of your sleep. Those living in climates without a lot of sun can use bright light therapy using a light box which will do the trick.

Serotonin is used to manage stress. The more stress you experience, the lower your levels of serotonin will be. Try to limit the stress in your lifestyle.

Positive thoughts increase your serotonin levels. Having a negative attitude and low self esteem can cause depression and lower your serotonin levels. If you are severely depressed, the doctor can prescribe a medication called Selective Serotonin Re-uptake Inhibitor (SSRI). If you're just feeling blue, then anti depressant medications tend not to work as well. Instead try natural remedies such as St John's Wort or SAM-E.

Make sure you are getting enough vitamin D. Deficiencies are common in colder climates, but even in sunny parts of the world, increased use of sunblock can decrease our absorption of vitamin D. A simple blood test can tell you if you need more of this vitamin. Supplements are cheap and easily available.

Certain foods contain serotonin, however the levels are quite low and don't make any difference to the levels in the brain. Of all the above advice, sunlight (or bright light therapy) probably offers the best solution.

There is a medication called **Sodium Oxybate** which has approved for sufferers of narcolepsy - a neurological sleep disorder- that may be beneficial for fibromyalgia sufferers. Sodium oxybate binds with GABA receptors in the brain to slow certain brain activity - namely slowing the fight or flight response - for up to four hours. Testing of this medication on fibromyalgia patients has produced a marked improvement in deep sleep quality, fatigue and pain levels. Speak to your doctor about Sodium oxybate to see if it may be suitable for you.

What on Earth is Phytotherapy?

The simple explanation for phytotherapy is the use of herbs to heal the body. Although herbal remedies have been in use for many years, there is still a lot of confusion that surrounds their use.

This is mainly because herbs have not been studied in the same ways as medications. They have not been through the rigorous testing process that all medications have to go through. However just because western medication has been deemed safe, this doesn't always mean that it is.

Herbal remedies have been used since the beginning of time to cure various ailments, however this does not mean that these remedies are not potent. Herbal remedies can be very effective, but can also negatively react with any medication you may be taking. Always discuss with your doctor any herbal remedies before starting.

Also keep in mind that phytotherapy is not a quick fix. Give the treatments time to do their work. They are giving the body the means to heal itself and this doesn't happen overnight.

Some of the herbs I have mentioned below are anti-inflammatory. There is divided opinion on whether fibromyalgia is an inflammatory disease or not. However the anti-inflammatory herbs do have other health benefits. Give them a try and if you notice no improvement in around twelve weeks, they're probably not going to help.

St John's Wort

This is the herbalist's answer to Prozac and a lot less addictive. If you're feeling depressed, a cup of St John's Wort tea may be just what you need. St John's Wort is also beneficial for sleep problems, having a calming effect. This herb also has anti inflammatory properties.

5HTP is a precursor for serotonin and is almost a must for those with fibromyalgia. It decreases pain levels and helps sleep. I have written more about 5HTP in the Central Sensitization chapter.

SAM-E is another way to increase your serotonin levels. More on SAM-E is the diet chapter.

Turmeric

This is a bright yellow spice with a considerable array of health benefits. It reduces pain and inflammation in fibromyalgia and is a potent antioxidant. Turmeric acts in a similar way to bromelain. It is an anti- inflammatory herb for fibromyalgia, as well as a pain reducer and blood thinner.

Valerian root, Passionflower, Skullcap and Hops. I have grouped these herbs together as they are all beneficial for those who have trouble sleeping. You can take them separately or together. They are quite often found together in some OTC herbal sleep remedies as they tend to have a synergistic effect.

Ginkgo Biloba is a herb that has been proven beneficial to fibromyalgia sufferers, especially when take in conjunction with CoQ10.

Ginger is a root which is used a lot in cooking and typically associated with travel sickness. However ginger can benefit those with fibromyalgia. It contains a digestive enzyme called Zingibain which will help digest proteins and calm the intestines. Ginger is also an anti-spasmodic which eases muscle cramps and relieves pain. Eat as much ginger as you like, there are no side effects.

Does Fascia Matter?

There has been a lot of talk on natural health sites and in forums on the importance of fascia in fibromyalgia. Fascia is the fibrous sheath that surrounds all the muscles in the body and tapers off towards the end of the muscle to form a tendon that attaches the muscles to the skeleton.

Speculation has it that the fascia has nerves and is capable of feeling pain. There is also a lot of talk about the fascia becoming tight and compressing the muscles to the point where pain is felt.

So what role does fascia play in fibromyalgia and should we be concerned about it?

Apart from supporting muscles and attaching them to the bones, the main purpose of fascia is to prevent infections from entering the body, especially after the body has been wounded in any way. Fascia is a physical barrier and forms a second line of defense after the skin. If the fascia itself is damaged, whether through physical injury or simply a structural imbalance in the body, it attempts to self repair.

As fascia repairs it can form scar tissue which renders it more rigid than before, hence the theory that this could cause fibromyalgia pain. There is also a theory that inflammation of the fascia can also cause central sensitization which is discussed more in the Central Sensitization chapter. Central sensitization causes fibromyalgia patients to experience pain differently to normal individuals and also increases pain signals to the brain.

To counteract this, there is a type of massage therapy known as myofacial release therapy (MRT) that has evolved which claims to release tight spots in the fascia so that it no longer causes fibromyalgia pain. This is also related to trigger point therapy or myofacial trigger point therapy.

While this all sounds good in theory, the fact is that fascia is an extremely tough substance and is not easily manipulated. While there are claims of people who have experienced MRT and have had significant pain reduction, this is probably not so much because the fascia has been released as it is because the tightness in the muscles has been relieved.

MRT is a deep tissue massage that is very intense, hence it's not suitable for everyone. There have been reports of injury as a result of MRT in extreme cases. The truth is, fascia can't be manipulated to the point of stretching it or making it more pliable. By all means try deep tissue massage if you think it may help, but make sure the therapist doesn't use excessive force. Always drink plenty of water and rest after this type of massage.

So if fascia can't be manipulated sufficiently to make any beneficial changes, is there anything that can be done to make it more comfortable and heal any potential scarring?

Stretching can benefit both fascia and muscles and can be done daily to relieve tightness. Make sure you warm up for at least ten minutes before stretching to prevent muscle injury. You will receive much more benefit from stretching when your muscles are warm.

Make sure you have adequate magnesium in your diet to prevent muscle tightness from magnesium deficiency.

Scarring in any part of the body may be relieved by taking a good proteolytic enzyme supplement on an empty stomach (between meals) three times a day. The Serrapeptase in the supplement will attack fibrin (scar tissue) and help remove it from the body. Proteolytic enzymes will also prevent chronic inflammation and block the release of pain inducing chemicals from inflamed tissues.

Whether or not fascia contributes to F pain is a moot point as little can be done to manipulate fascia. Fascia is too tough to stretch with manual manipulation and is probably made that way for a reason.

False are the main claims of fascial release therapy, which primarily concerns correcting postural asymmetries, eliminating alleged restrictions, and treating chronic pain.

Paul Ingraham - http://saveyourself.ca/articles/does-fascia-matter.php -

Conclusion

I hope you have found this book helpful in decreasing your fibromyalgia symptoms. Remember that natural treatments, unlike drugs, do take a while to work, so give them a few weeks before trying something else.

Fibromyalgia is a complex mix of different symptoms, so needs a complex approach. It could almost be described as the body's rejection of the 21st century lifestyle. So anything that will relieve the chemical load on the body is bound to help, whether this be food, personal care items and mental or physical stress.

A positive attitude, while hard to achieve, will definitely help. There is absolutely a mind-body connection.

If this book has helped you, I would really appreciate you going to Amazon and leaving a review.

I wish you the best of health!

Further recommended reading...
Fibromyalgia: A Guide to Understanding the Journey
What Your Doctor May Not Tell You About Fibromyalgia
The Fatigue and Fibromyalgia Solution

Wendy Owen's other books in the Natural Health Books Series...
Type 2 Diabetes Cure
Rheumatoid Arthritis Pain Relief

Disclaimer

The author is not a medical doctor or a practitioner in the conventional medical field.

The information in this book is provided for informational purposes only and is not a substitute for professional medical advice. The author makes no legal claims, express or implied. Readers are advised to do their own due diligence when it comes to making medical decisions and the material here provided is not intended to replace the advice of a qualified physician.

The author assumes no responsibility for the loss or damage caused, or allegedly caused, directly or indirectly by the use of information contained in this book. The author and publisher specifically disclaim any liability incurred from the use or application of the contents of this book.

No part of this book may be reproduced or transmitted in any form by any means, electronic, mechanical, photocopying, recording, or otherwise, without the prior written permission of the author. The information and opinions expressed in this publication are believed to be accurate and sound, based on the information available to the author.

Printed in Great Britain
by Amazon